MEDICAL ROBOTS

LUKE COLINS

BLACK RABBIT BOOKS

Bolt Jr. is published by Black Rabbit Books
P.O. Box 3263, Mankato, Minnesota, 56002.
www.blackrabbitbooks.com

Catherine Cates, interior designer; Grant Gould, cover designer; Omay Ayres, photo researcher

Names: Colins, Luke, author.
Title: Medical robots / by Luke Colins.
Description: Mankato, Minnesota : Black Rabbit Books, [2020] | Series: Bolt Jr. World of robots | Includes bibliographical references and index. |
Audience: Age 6-8. | Audience: K to Grade 3.
Identifiers: LCCN 2019001937 (print) | LCCN 2019002716 (ebook) | ISBN 9781623101701 (ebook) | ISBN 9781623101640 (library binding) | ISBN 9781644661086 (paperback)
Subjects: LCSH: Robotics in medicine—Juvenile literature. | Robots—Juvenile literature. | Medical technology—Juvenile literature. | Medical innovations—Juvenile literature.
Classification: LCC R857.R63 (ebook) | LCC R857.R63 C65 2020 (print) | DDC 610.285—dc23
LC record available at https://lccn.loc.gov/2019001937

Printed in the United States. 5/19

Image Credits

Getty: JIJI PRESS, 16–17; Shutterstock: ALIENFORCE, 18–19 (bkgd); Andrey Suslov, Cover; Christos Georghiou, 10–11 (body); Ivan Chudakov, 8–9; kung_tom, 6–7; Lightspring, 20–21; Martin Nezval, 3, 24; Meganeura, 10 (face); Motionblur Studios, 7; Ociacia, 8; Phonlamai Photo, 18–19 (bot), 22–23; ProStockStudio, 14–15 (bkgd); Vinne, 12; Volodymyr Horbovyy, 4, 21; whitehoune, 1, 13; Superstock: Javier Larrea / age fotostock, 5

Contents

CHAPTER 1

Helpful Bots

A man lies on the table. Robot arms move toward his **heart**. A doctor tells the arms where to go. Together, the doctor and robot fix the heart.

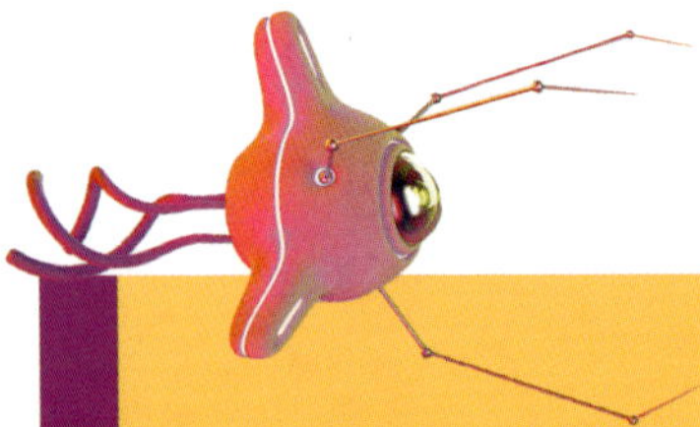

heart: an organ that moves blood in the body

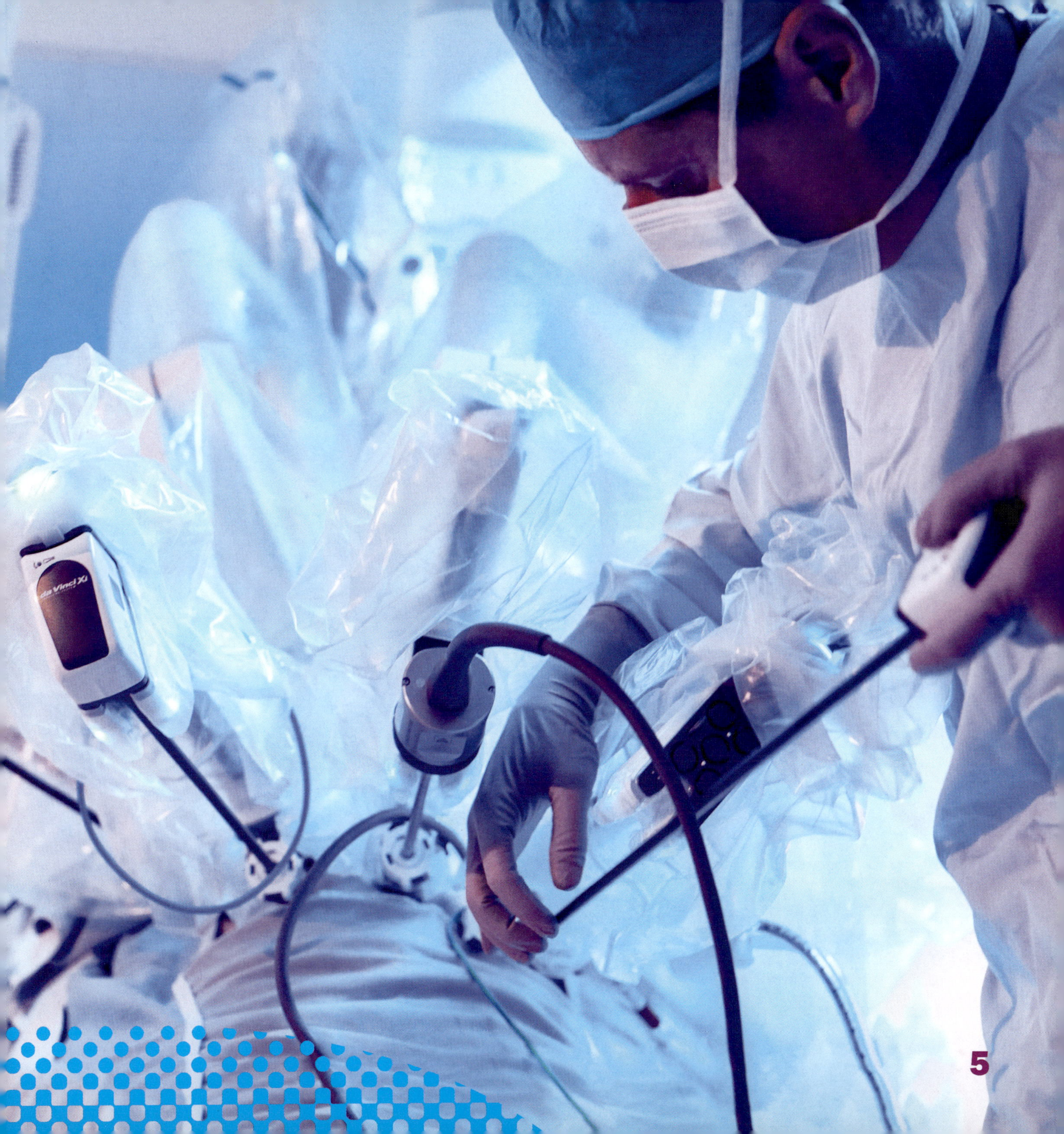
da Vinci Xi

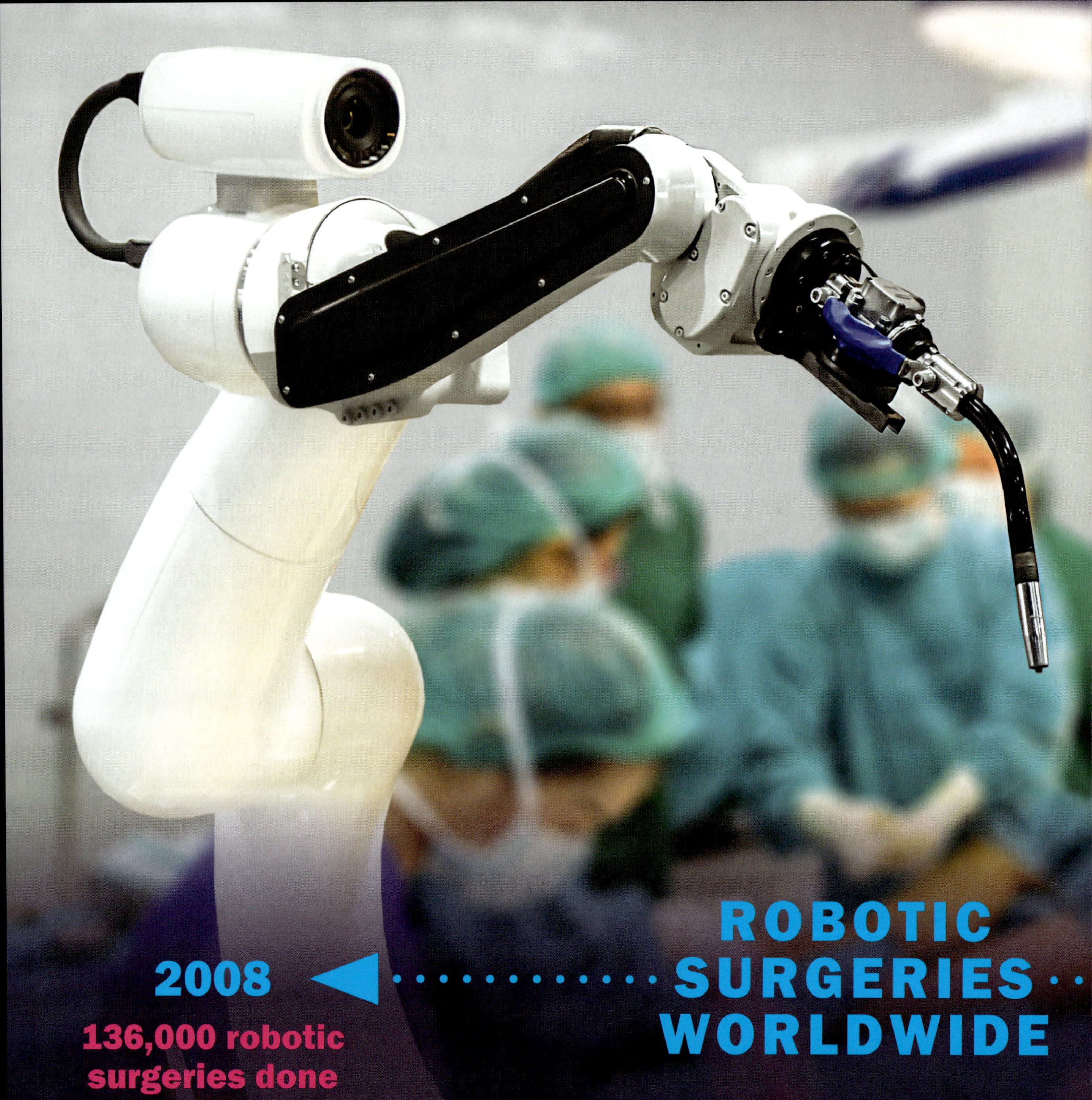

ROBOTIC SURGERIES WORLDWIDE

2008

136,000 robotic surgeries done

Cool Helpers

Around the world, doctors use robots. Bots help in surgeries. Others bring supplies. People even wear some bots.

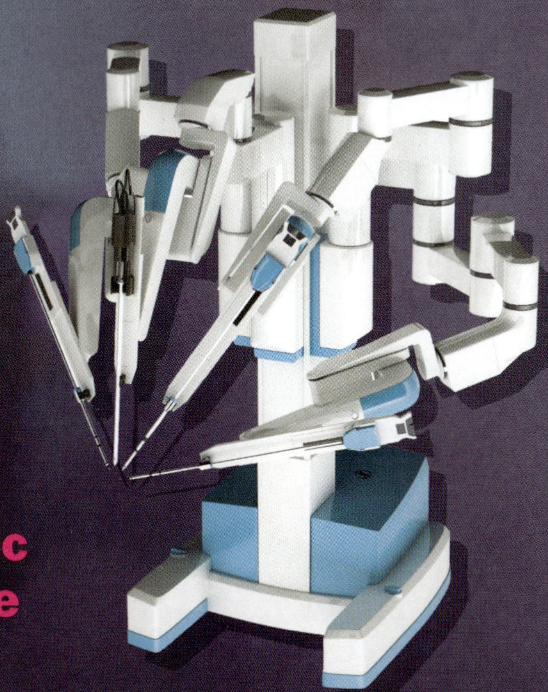

2017

877,000 robotic surgeries done

CHAPTER 2

Wearing Bots

People use many medical robots. Some go in the body. People wear others. Robotic legs help people walk. Robot eyes help **blind** people see.

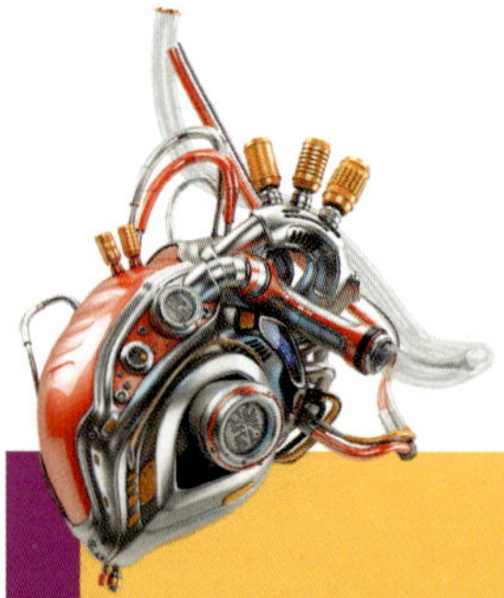

blind: unable to see

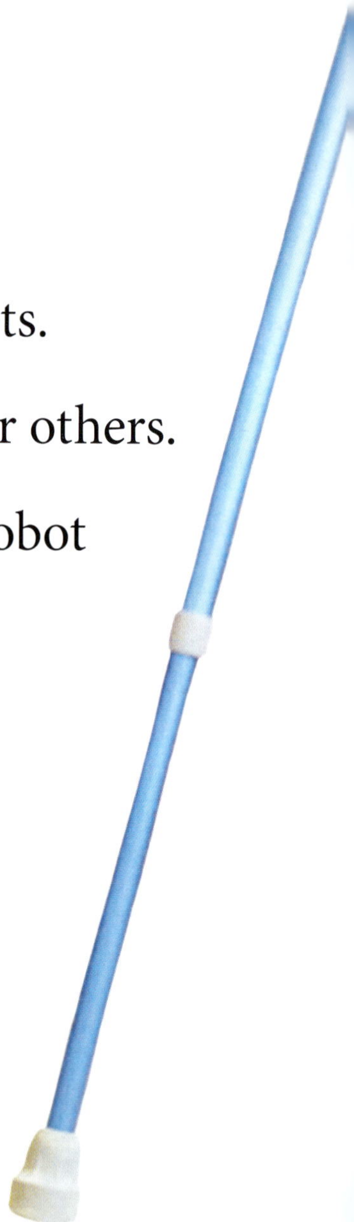

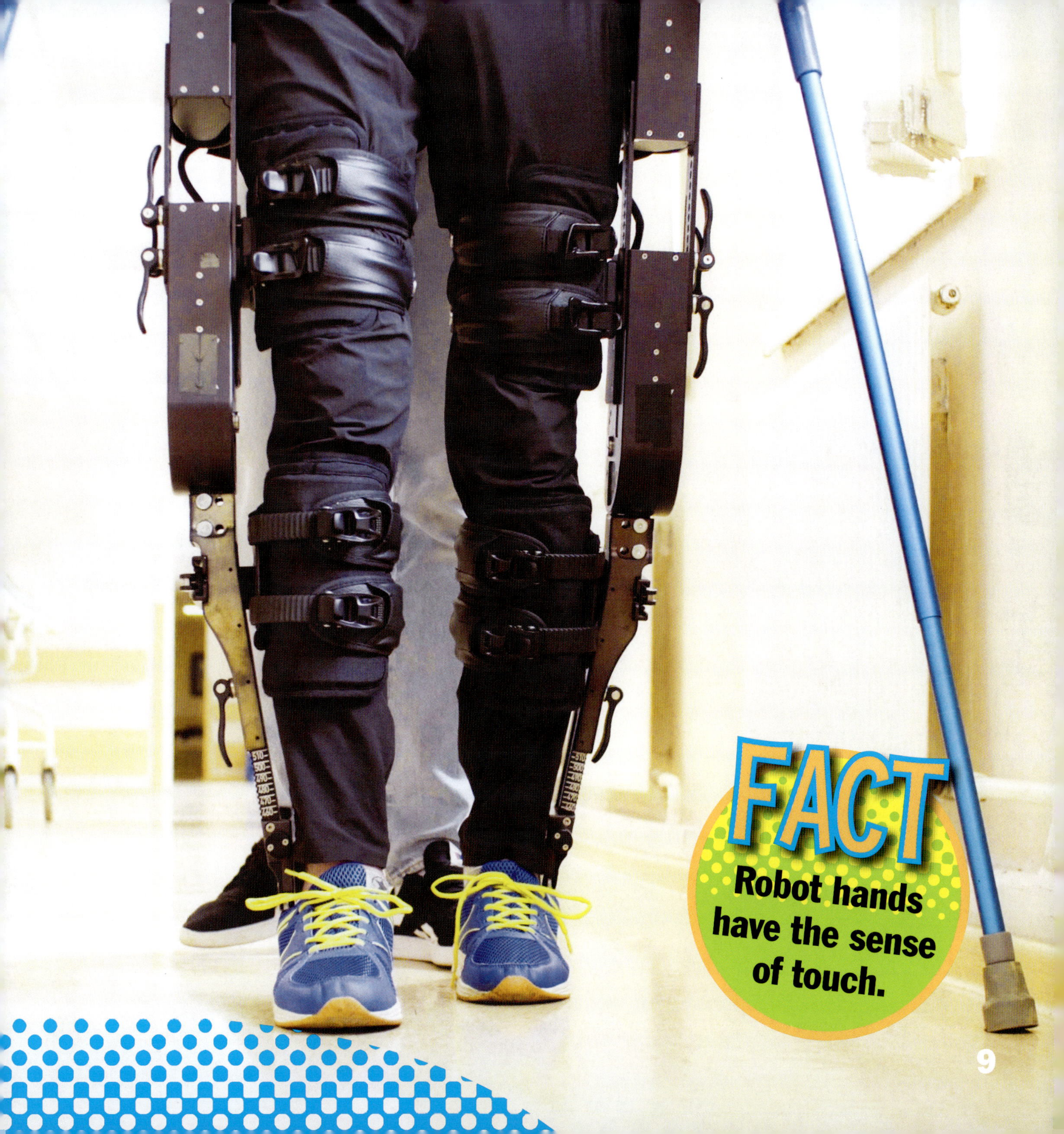

FACT

Robot hands have the sense of touch.

WHERE BOTS HAVE BEEN USED

On the Body

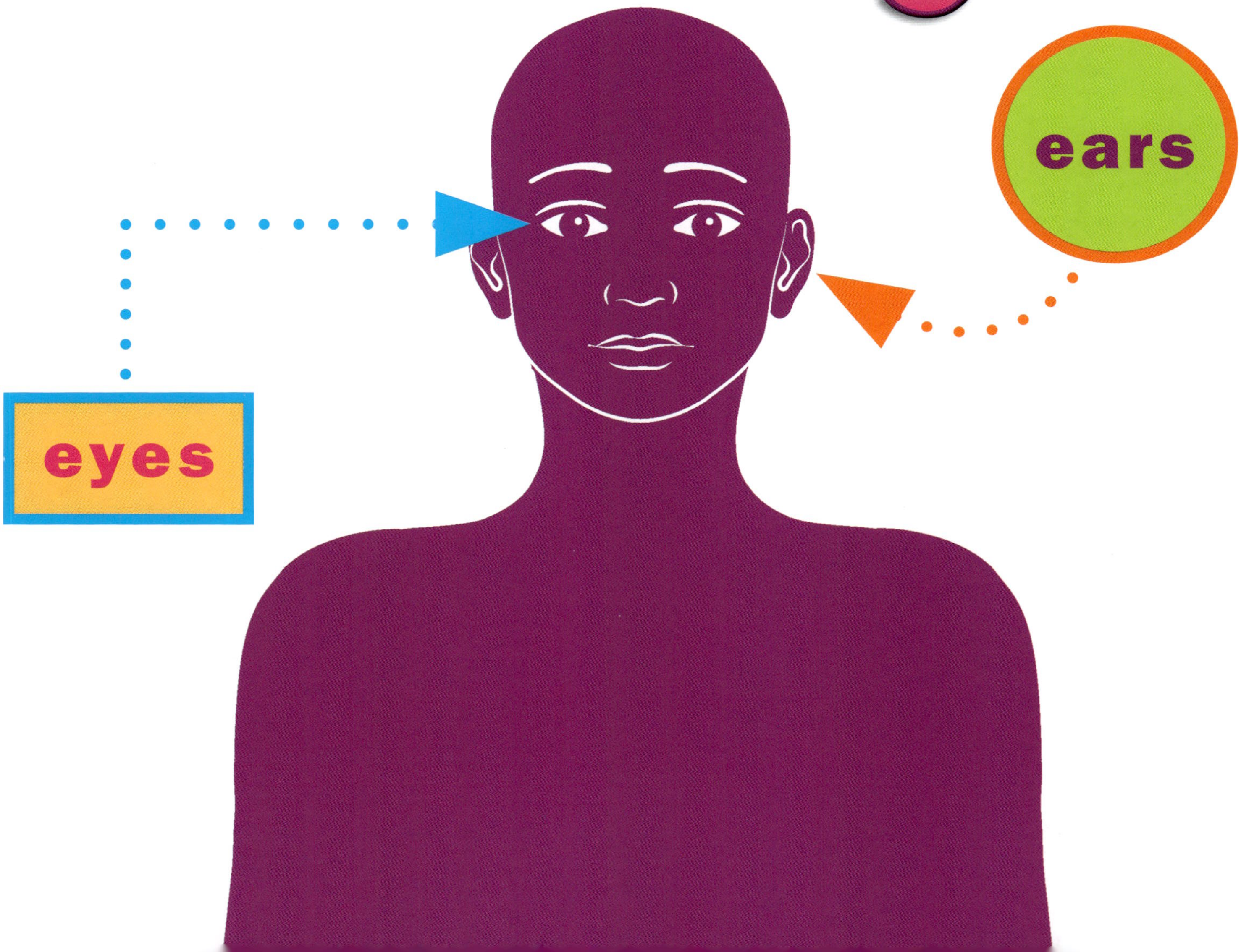

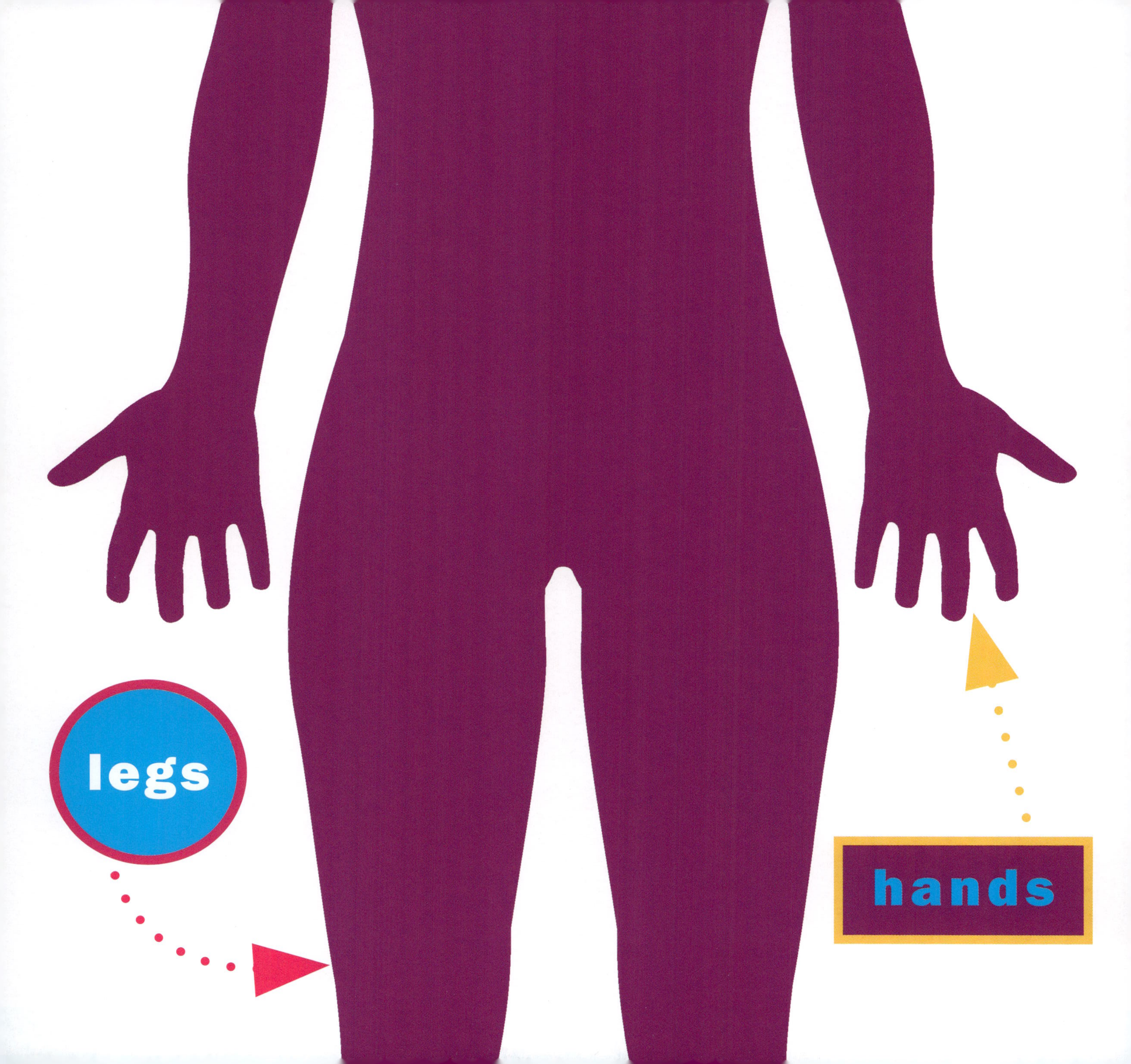
legs
hands

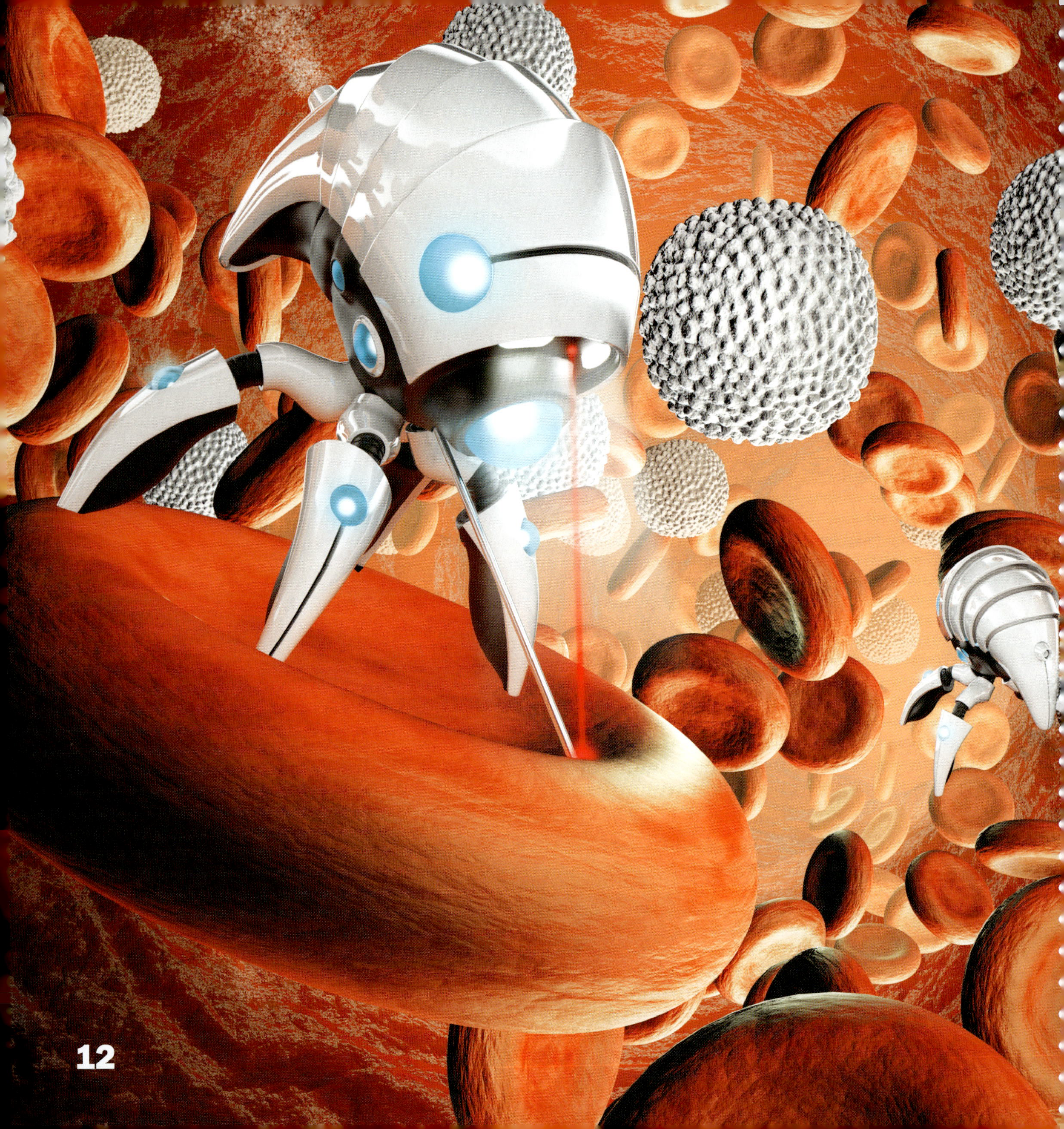

Deep Inside

Some tiny bots are used inside people. These bots move in the blood. Some carry medicine. Others clear **blocked** spots.

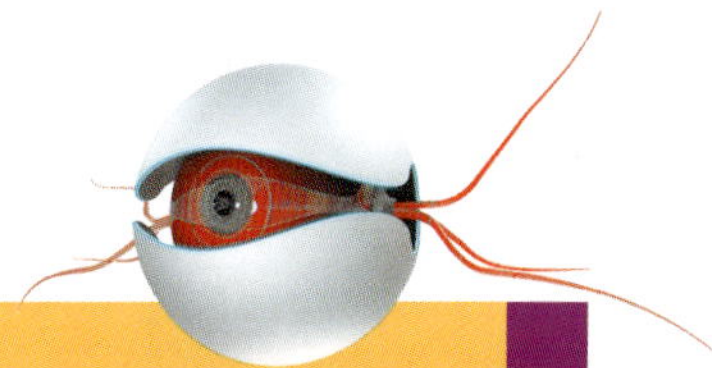

blocked: closed off by something

Where Most Robotic Surgeries Are Done

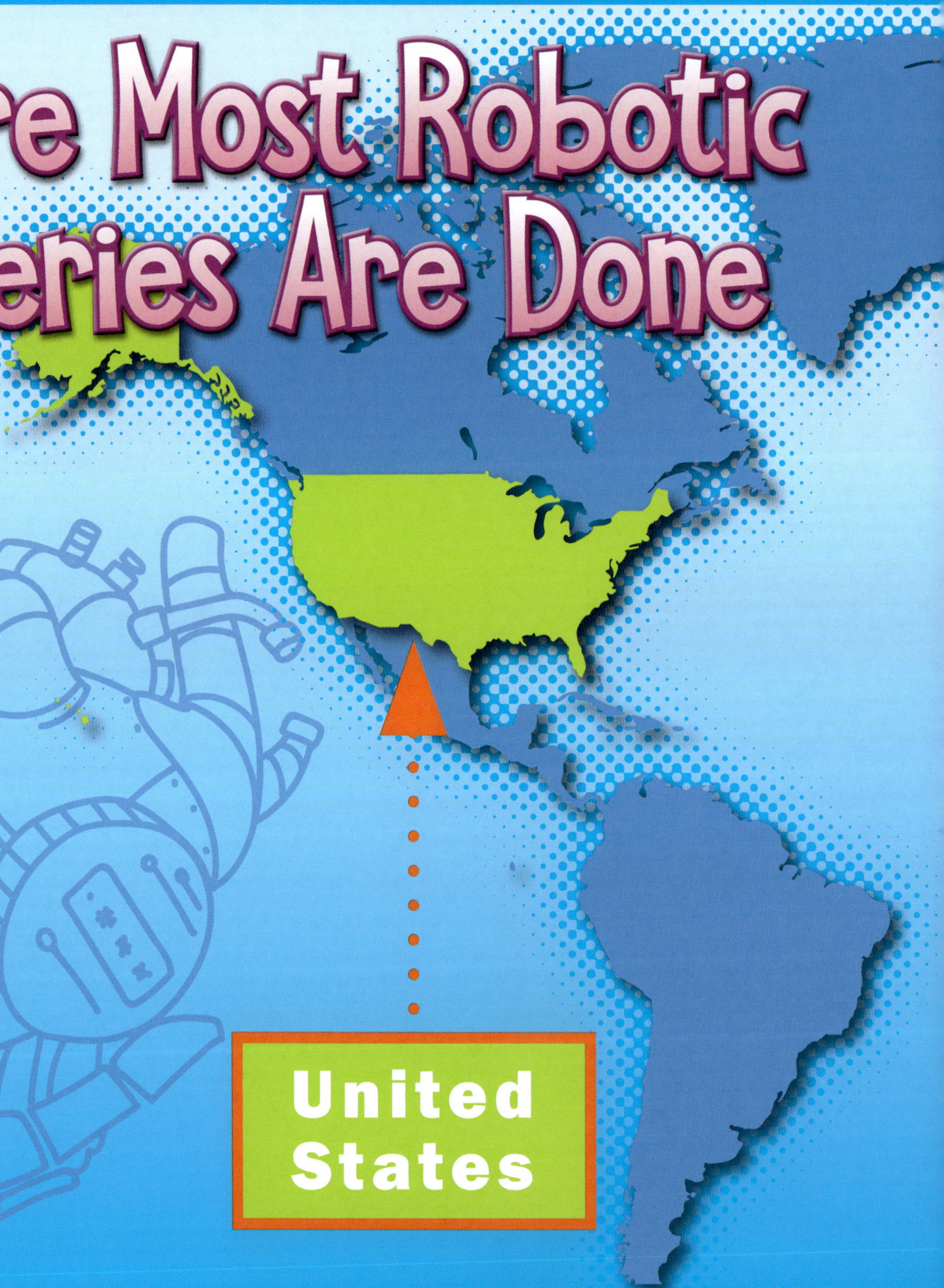

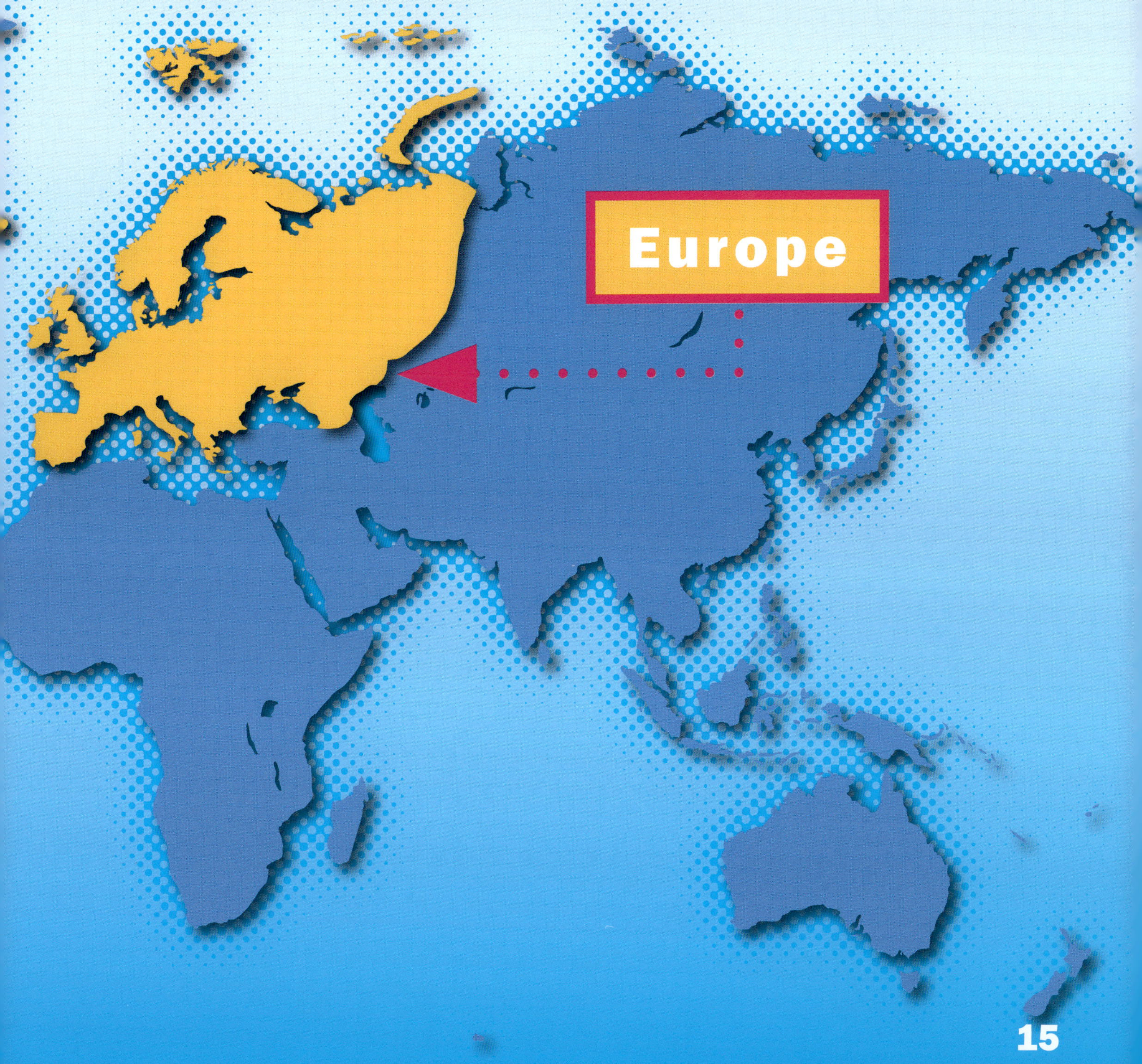
Europe

CHAPTER 3

Hospital Helpers

Medical bots have jobs too. Some bots lift people from bed. Others open doors. Another kind carries medicine.

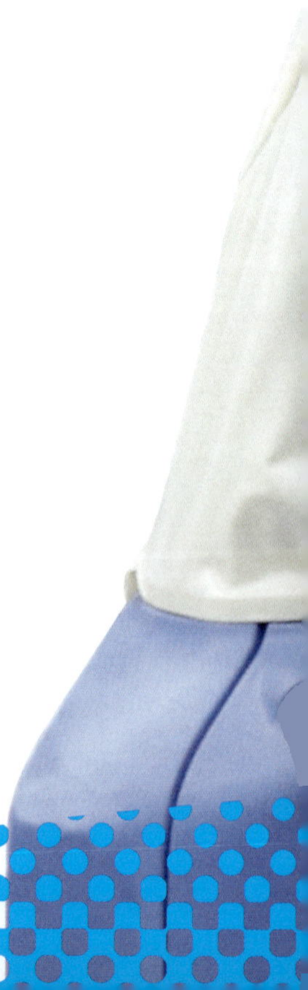

FACT

Another bot helps people exercise.

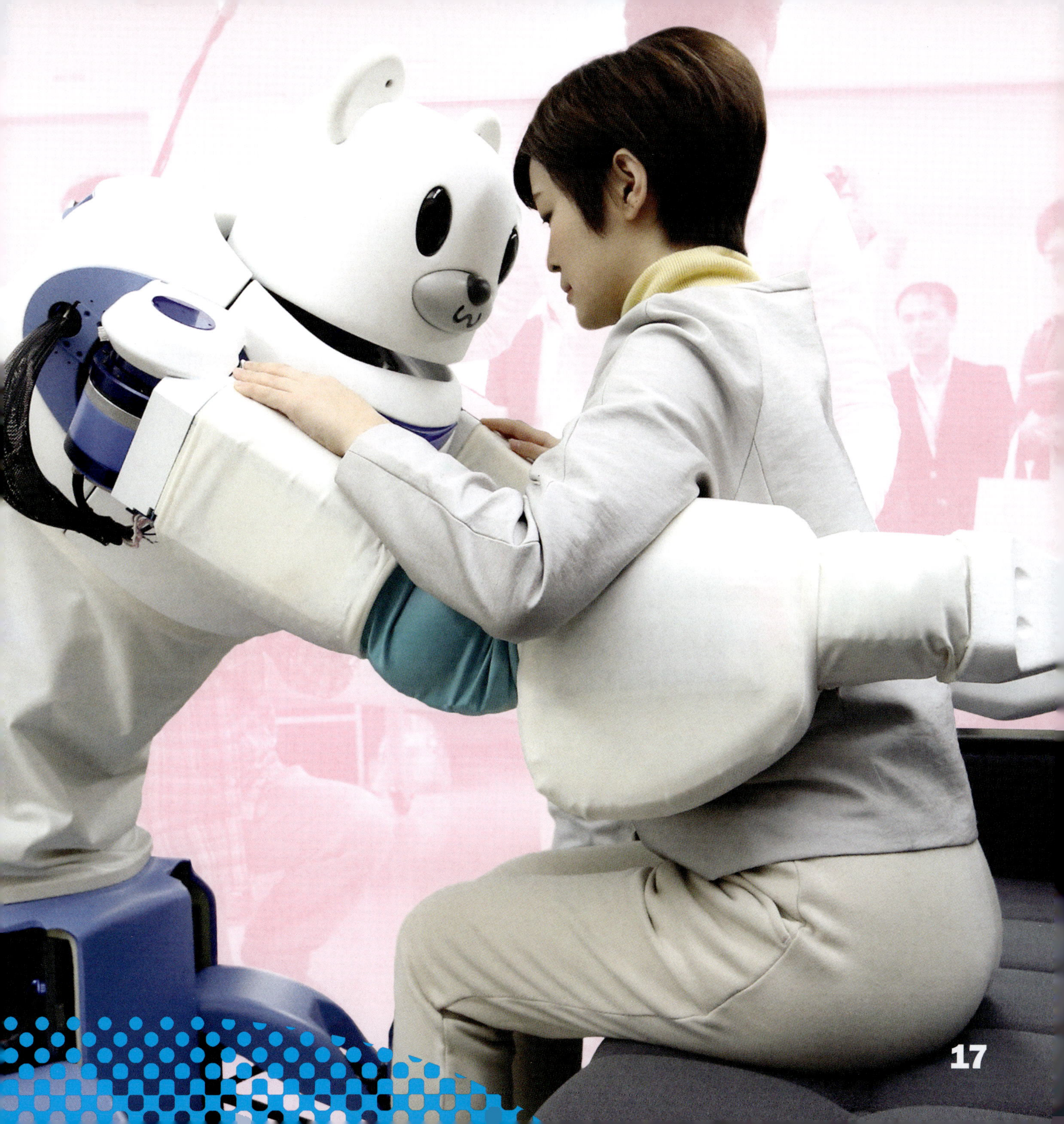

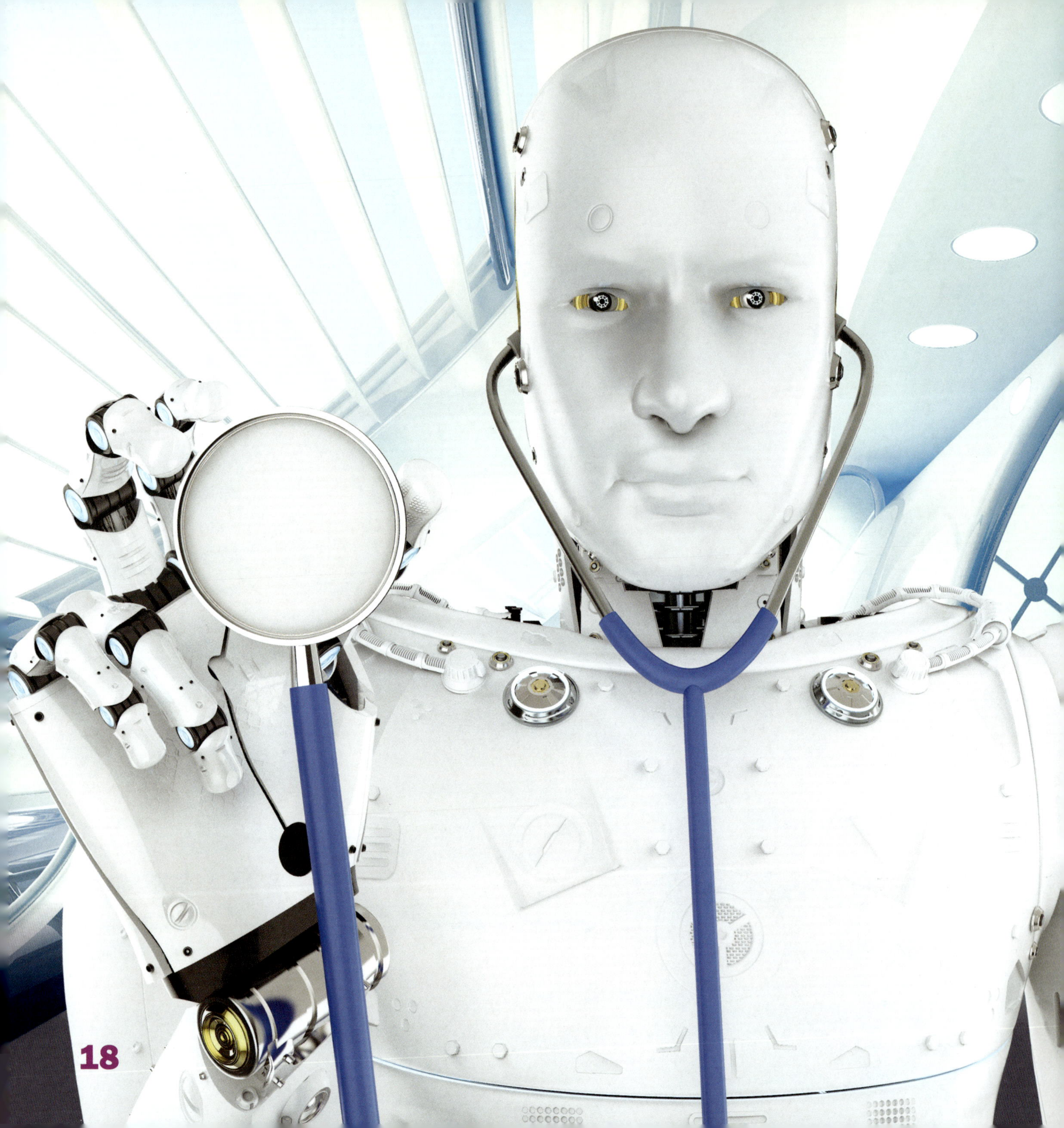

The Future

Robots help in many ways. Scientists are making new bots. Maybe one day, bots will be the doctors. What do you think?

Growing Use

Hospitals might spend $18 billion on robots by 2024.

Bonus Facts

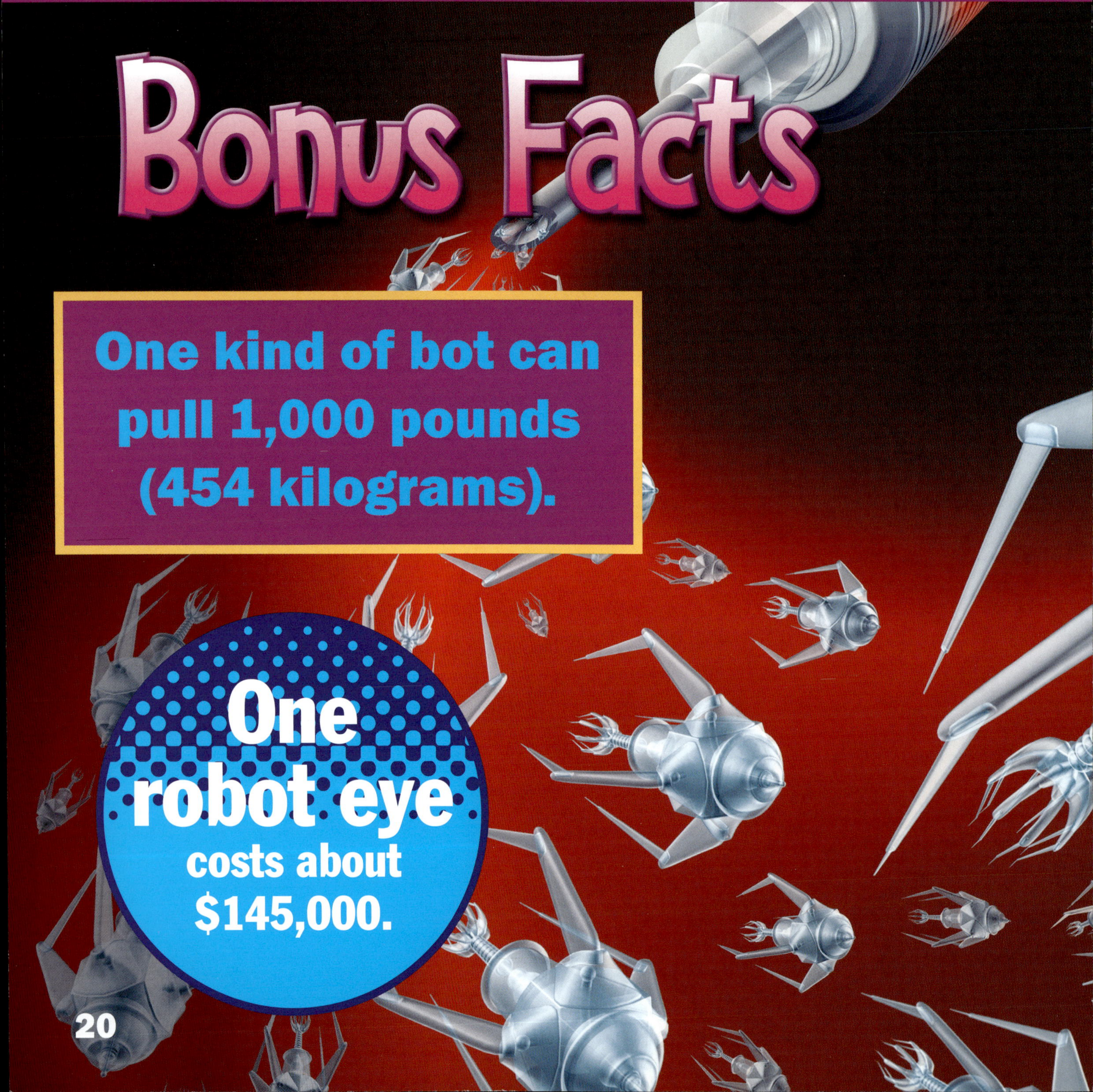

One kind of bot can pull 1,000 pounds (454 kilograms).

One robot eye costs about $145,000.

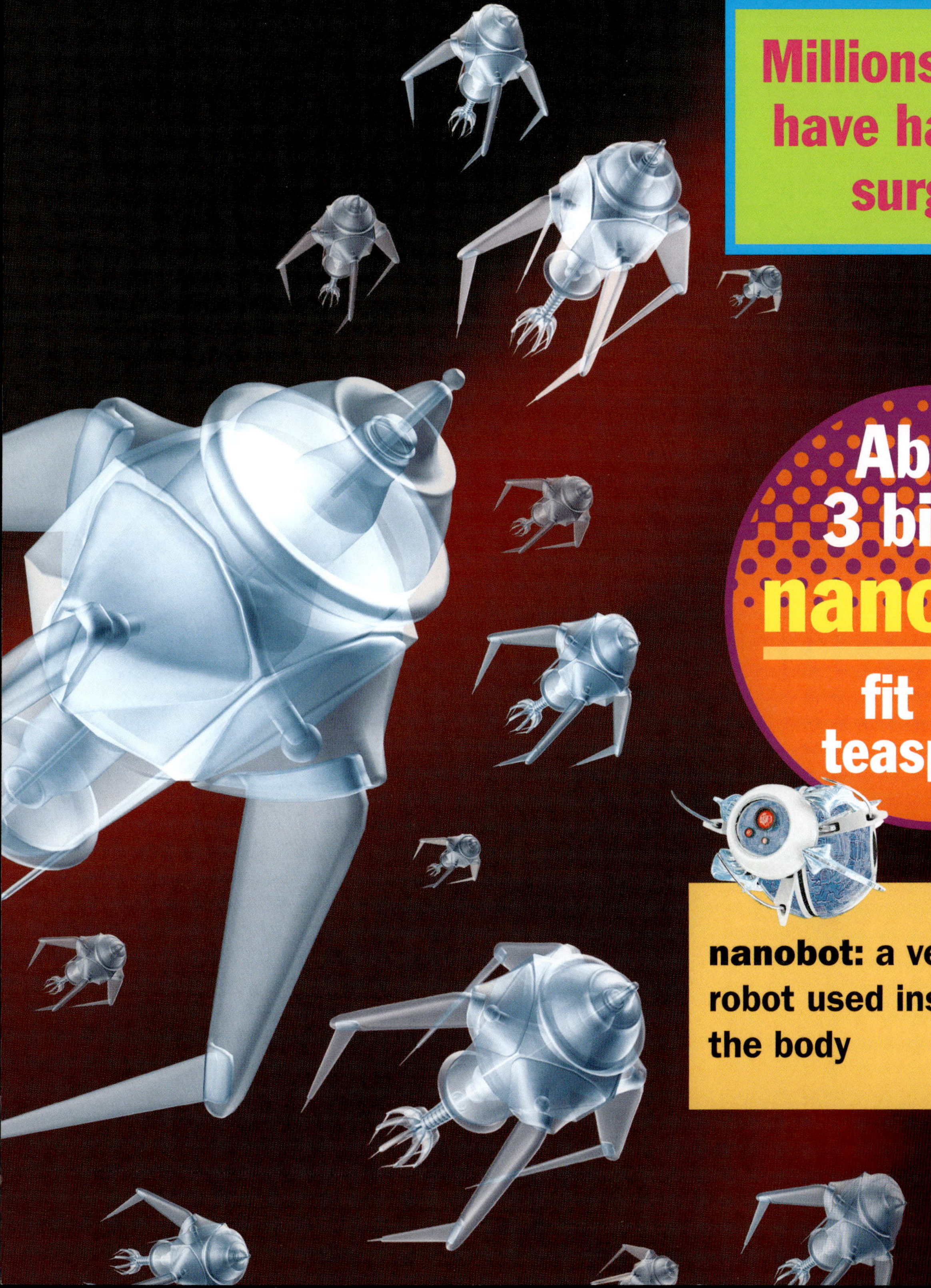

Millions of people have had robotic surgeries.

About 3 billion nanobots fit in a teaspoon.

nanobot: a very tiny robot used inside the body

READ MORE/WEBSITES

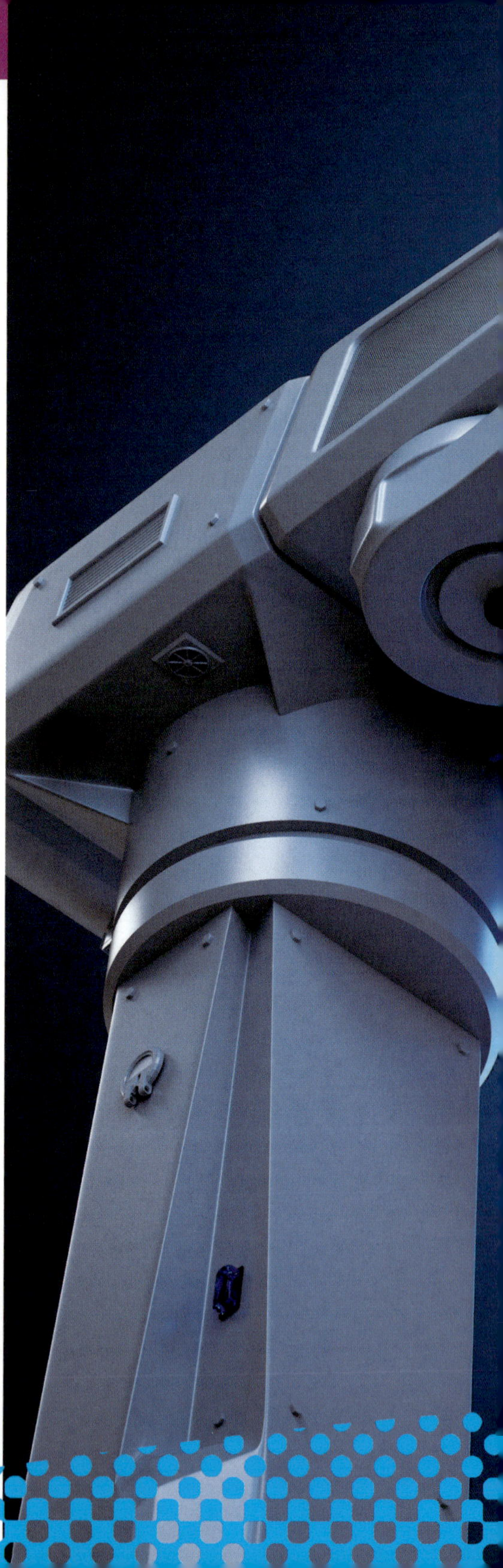

Higgins, Nadia. *Medical Robots.* Robotics in Our World. Mankato, MN: Amicus High Interest/Amicus Ink, 2018.

Kelly, John. *Fixer the Robot.* London: Faber & Faber, 2018.

Latta, Sara L. *Zoom in on Medical Robots.* Zoom in on Robots. New York: Enslow Publishing, 2018.

Robotics
kidsahead.com/subjects/1-robotics

Robotics: Facts
idahoptv.org/sciencetrek/topics/robots/facts.cfm

Robots for Kids
sciencekids.co.nz/robots.html

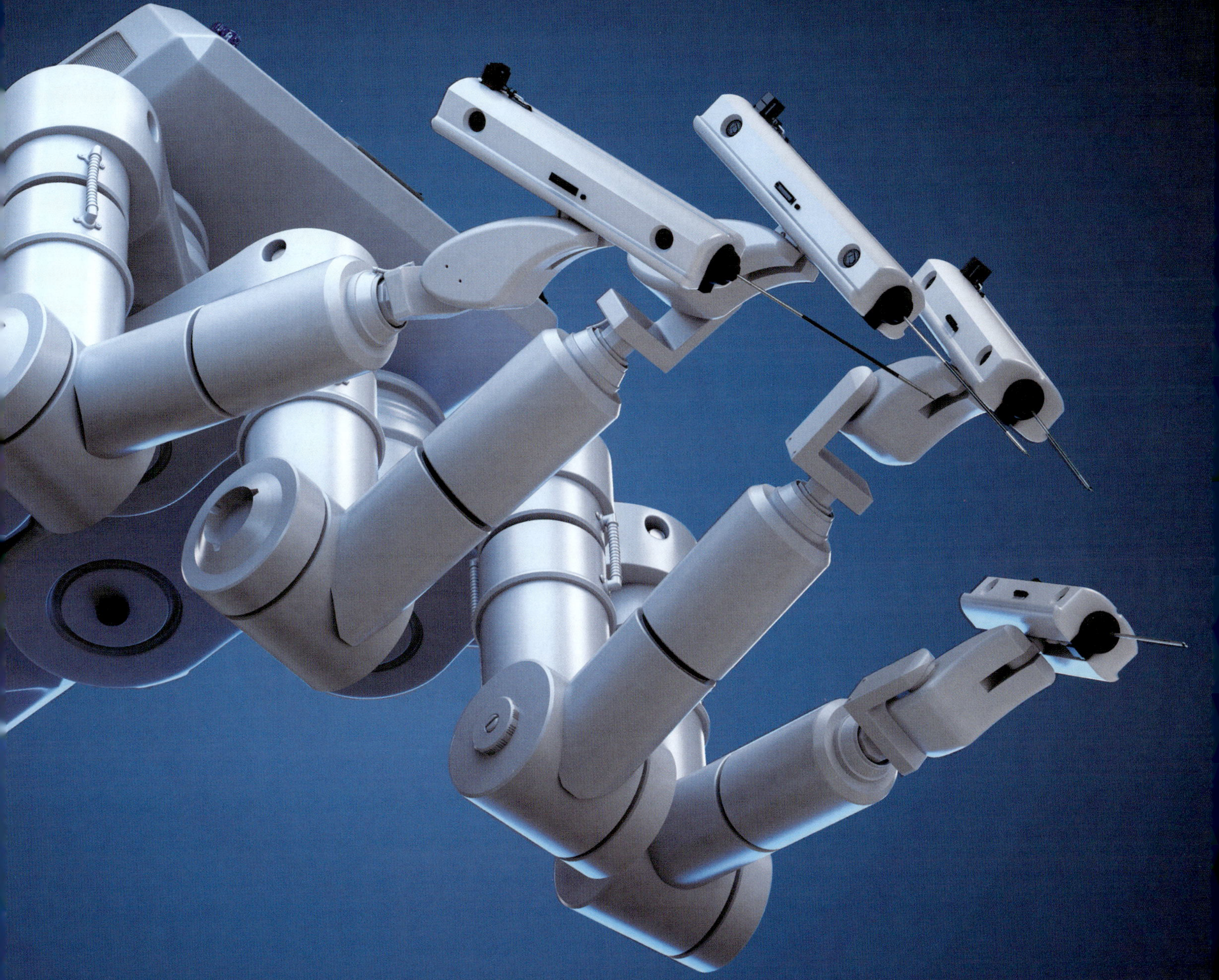

GLOSSARY

blind (BLIND)—unable to see

blocked (BLAHKT)—closed off by something

heart (HART)—an organ that moves blood in the body

nanobot (NAH-no-baht)—a very tiny robot used inside the body

INDEX